Copyright © 2014 Christie Knight

All rights reserved. No part of this publi or distributed in any form or by any mea or retrieval system, without the prior written permission... author, except where permitted by law.

Legal & Disclaimer

The information contained in this book is not designed to replace or take the place of any form of medication or professional medical advice. The information in this book has been provided for educational and entertainment purposes only.

The information contained in this book has been compiled from sources deemed reliable, and it is accurate to the best of the Author's knowledge. However, the Author cannot guarantee its accuracy and validity so cannot be held liable for any errors or omissions. Changes are periodically made to this book. You must consult your doctor or get professional medical advice before using any of the suggested remedies, techniques, or information in this book.

Upon using the information contained in this book, you agree to hold harmless the Author from and against any damages, costs and expenses, including any legal fees, potentially resulting from the application of any of the information provided by this guide. This disclaimer applies to any damages or injury caused by the use and application, whether directly or indirectly, of any advice or information presented, whether for breach of contract, tort, negligence, personal injury, criminal intent, or under any other cause of action.

You agree to accept all the risks of using the information presented inside this book. You need to consult a professional medical practitioner in order to ensure you are both able & healthy enough to participate in this program.

Contents

Introduction 4

Chapter 1 Nurture Yourself and Your Unborn Baby 6
   Foods That Nurture You and Baby's Brain.............................. 7
   Healthy and Delicious Recipes.. 8
   Foods of Great Nutritional Value 11
   Music 12

Chapter 2 Ways to Cope With the Physical and Emotional Aspects of Pregnancy.. 13
   Common Ailments.. 14
   Prenatal Yoga.. 16

Chapter 3 Pregnancy Myths 19
   Myth 1 20
   Myth 2 20
   Myth 3 21
   Myth 4 21
   Myth 5 21
   Myth 6 21
   Myth 7 22

Chapter 4 Childbirth Options That Work for You 23
   The development of the baby 25
   Get Ready For Baby!.. 26

Chapter 5 What to Expect 30 Days After......................... 29
   Recognizing Postpartum Depression (PPD)........................ 31
   How to treat PPD 31
   Learn How Babies Communicate.. 33

Soothing Newborn Colic *33*
Hours of sleep for newborn *34*

Chapter 6 Breastfeed or Formula Feed 36

Bonus Material 45

Conclusion 50

Introduction

Introduction here Congrats on your pregnancy! It may come as a shock or surprise and can be both great and scary news! Either way, these are exciting times. Now you get the real fun of letting your family, friends, and coworkers know. Of course, you know what comes along with that: a lot of fussing and belly rubbing.

Your baby has already begun to grow, which starts the body into a subtle tizzy of changes for the next nine months. Not all women experience morning sickness, but don't be surprised if certain smells or foods make you nauseous. You might begin to feel sick or fatigued from simple tasks. From here on, expect to gain at least one pound a week. Before you know it, you will be carrying around a basketball in your shirt and will soon be counting down the days of when the baby will finally arrive. Until then, take it one step at a time, and try your best to bond with your baby while he or she is still in the womb.

The next chapter will give you a glimpse into what to expect in the next nine months of pregnancy (as much as can be predicted!). This book can be used as a tool to help you decide which delivery options will work best for you, and it also offers natural options on how to cope with your changing body. You will also be given plenty of organic options to nurture both yourself and your baby on all physical, mental, and emotional planes.

Natural remedies for common symptoms save stress, time, and money. Holistic answers, like aromatherapy and healthy eating, are consistent and non-evasive ways to make your pregnancy go as smoothly and naturally as possible. Organic and natural answers for common ailments for both baby and mommy are also mentioned in this book. You will also get a glimpse of things to expect up to birth, delivery, and the first thirty days after.

We will discuss the facts behind many of the myths that come along with pregnancy. We are all told during our pregnancy that we should not do certain things or eat certain foods, but we have to educate ourselves about which is fact and which is fiction.

Not everything can be predictable when expecting a baby, but knowing the basics definitely helps.

Happy motherhood!

Chapter 1
Nurture Yourself and Your Unborn Baby

Chapter 1: Nurture Yourself and Your Unborn Baby

While researching this book, I found a common gripe. Most pregnancy books all want their reader moms to be perfect. Don't even think about eating unhealthy foods. Don't even think about donuts, or ice cream, or pie, or slushies. That is way too much pressure! Listen, if you are craving for something, it might be for a very good reason. Of course, as a general rule of thumb, don't forget about your nutritious foods too.

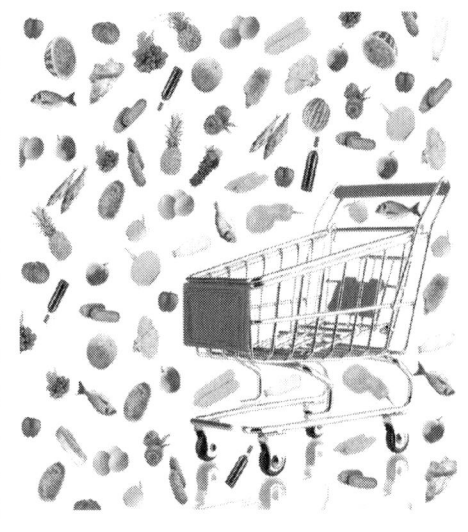

See a health care professional as soon as possible after you find out that you're pregnant. You can now start thinking about scheduling checkups and talking to your doctors about prenatal vitamins. Aside from those, you (when the cravings aren't making you crazy) will most likely feel the need to treat your body better than usual, since there is an entire other person growing inside you.

Foods That Nurture You and Baby's Brain

For starters, don't be afraid to choose bacon! Research has shown that eating pork and eggs helps to develop the brain cells of an unborn baby. Studies also show the benefits that eating fish has on both mom's and baby's brains. Eating fish twice a week can help improve the unborn baby's language and motor skills. But, you need to be cautious of the fish you will be eating. Make sure you do not eat fish that have high mercury levels, which isn't good for the baby.

However, don't let this intimidate your fish eating adventures! Fish is loaded with omega-3 fatty acids and is crucial for developing baby's eyes, brain, and entire nervous system. It also carries qualities that give you lots of natural energy, which you will definitely need, and is full of vitamin D and protein.

Your safest bet is to stay away from larger, more predatory fish like sharks, swordfish, king mackerel, and tilefish. Do your best not to exceed more than 12 ounces of fish a week, to ensure the healthiest mercury levels.

Here are a few types of fish that are safe to eat during pregnancy:

- Catfish
- Clams
- Cod
- Crab
- Flounder
- Haddock
- Herring
- Oysters (cooked)
- Pollock
- Rainbow Trout
- Salmon
- Sardine
- Shrimp
- Tilapia
- Whitefish

Healthy and Delicious Recipes

Recipe 1- The Ultimate Healthy Fish Recipe

It's called the ultimate because you can use this recipe with pretty much any type of fish listed above. Although white fillets, halibut, Pollock, and tilapia are favored.

You will need:

1 teaspoon of olive oil

½ pound of fresh, sliced mushrooms

½ pound of fresh, chopped spinach

¼ teaspoon crushed, oregano leaves

1 clove of garlic, minced

1 ½ pounds white fish fillet

2 tablespoons of orange juice

1 cup of grated mozzarella cheese

Olive oil

Cooking spray

Skillet

10x6 baking dish

Preheat oven to 400 degrees and spray the baking dish with cooking spray. Heat a small amount of olive oil in the skillet and sauté the mushrooms until tender (about three minutes), then add spinach. Continue sautéing until spinach is slightly wilted, then remove from heat. Drain juices from the skillet into the baking dish. Stir garlic and oregano in with the mushrooms and spinach.

Finally, place an even amount of the vegetables in the center of each fillet and place into the baking dish. Pour orange juice and sprinkle grated mozzarella cheese on top and bake for 15 to 20 minutes.

Recipe via

http://babyfit.sparkpeople.com/pregnancy-recipes.asp?id=322

Recipe 2- Delicious Chicken Dinner

A pregnant woman should have at least 60 grams of protein daily, and this should be no problem at all since this recipe is packed with 50 grams of protein.

You will need:

5 ounces of chicken strips or tenders

2 egg whites

2 tablespoons of breadcrumbs

1 tablespoon of Parmesan cheese

½ teaspoon of oregano

¼ teaspoon of dry mustard

¼ teaspoon of garlic powder

Begin by preheating your oven to 475 degrees. The next thing you will want to do is place the 2 egg whites in a bowl and mix them together well with a fork. In a second bowl, combine the breadcrumbs, Parmesan cheese, oregano, mustard, and garlic powder, ensuring that they are mixed well.

Spray your baking sheet with nonstick cooking spray. Dip each chicken tender into the egg white, and then roll it carefully in the breadcrumb mixture. Place the chicken on the baking sheet. Bake the tenders for 15 minutes. Serve with marinara sauce for dipping for a snack, or for a meal served with sweet potato fries and one cup of steamed broccoli drizzled with 1 teaspoon of olive oil and lemon juice to taste.

Recipe 3- Healthy Vegetarian Meal

You may not always crave meats or you may be a vegetarian, but either way, it is still important for you to ensure that you are getting all of the vitamins and minerals that you and your baby need.

You will need:

1 medium acorn squash

½ cup of chopped onions

1/2 cup of chopped mushrooms

1/3 cup white beans

1 garlic clove, chopped

1 cup cooked brown rice

1 tablespoon of pistachios, chopped

Begin by preheating your oven to 375 degrees and then spray your baking pan with nonstick cooking spray. Cut your squash in half and remove the seeds, then place cut-side down on the baking pan, and cook for about 45 minutes or until it is tender.

While the squash is cooking you can begin to prepare the filling. In a pan on top of the stove, you will want to sauté the onion, mushrooms, white beans, and garlic until softened or about 5 minutes.

After 5 minutes you will add the cup of brown rice as well as the pistachios, and mix it all together well. Continue cooking for about 1 minute.

Once the squash has finished cooking, you will scoop the brown rice mixture into the squash and top with the Parmesan cheese. Place this back into the oven and cook for 10 more minutes.

Foods of Great Nutritional Value

Of course, you're not always going to have all the time to prepare such a great meal for yourself. If you're lucky, you might have someone to do it for you! Well, for those days you are on the go or don't feel much like cooking, keep these foods in mind, too. Each of them holds a great nutritional value.

> Dairy- Dairy products like yogurt act as a natural probiotic, which will help keep your digestive system healthy and your bowel movements regular.
>
> Legumes- These are a great source of fiber and will also help keep your digestive system functioning comfortably.
>
> Eggs- As mentioned before, eggs are a wonderful source of protein. The best thing about adding eggs into your regular diet is that they contain a small portion of each essential vitamin you need.
>
> Broccoli- Broccoli contains plenty of important vitamins, helps the digestive system, and is full of antioxidants for both you and baby.

Pork and Beef- These are both heavily rich in iron, something vitally important during pregnancy.

Berries- Berries are chock full of vitamin C, an important vitamin needed to maintain a healthy immune system.

Whole grains- Whole grains are full of the essential vitamin B as well as plenty of fibers necessary to help with digestion.

Water- It's important to stay hydrated and drink lots of water every day. This can help with headaches, constipation, fatigue, and urinary tract infections.

Music

Studies have shown that sound can reach your baby in the womb. Playing relaxing music (especially classical) has been proven to stimulate baby's brain from the start and raise the intelligence level. Reading books out loud can also potentially affect his or her IQ and overall personality.

A great way to use music as a tool is to put on some calming, soft music at night when the baby won't stop kicking, tossing, and turning. Doing this while the baby is in the womb may prove to be a good soothing technique to continue when the baby is born and is having a fussy, restless night.

We will now proceed to the next chapter, to explore ways to cope with the physical and emotional aspects of pregnancy, which is an important element to a stress-free pregnancy when you embrace the changes in you.

Chapter 2
Ways to Cope With the Physical and Emotional Aspects of Pregnancy

Chapter 2: Ways to Cope With the Physical and Emotional Aspects of Pregnancy

It's hard to know what to expect when it comes to body changes. Every mother, of course, is different. The quicker you can accept your changing body, the easier your pregnancy will be. Eat healthy as much as you can, and take time out for a little light exercise or prenatal yoga. These will help with the physical as well as mental and emotional changes.

Common Ailments

Some things might become more enticing than usual while others may make you feel sick. This usually lasts for the first three months of pregnancy. While you may have your good days and your bad days, morning sickness can put a real damper on things and leave you feeling down for the count.

Morning sickness can come on at pretty much any time it wants to, so it doesn't have to be only in the morning. Aside from making sure you stay hydrated with water, ask your doctor about vitamin B. A great way to avoid nausea is to nibble on starchy foods, like rice, pasta, bread, pretzels, and crackers. Other things that help settle the stomach are ginger tea, peppermint, peppermint tea, and ginger ale.

Heartburn

One common way to avoid heartburn is to eat smaller meals, more frequently. Eating too fast and having an overly full stomach could lead to uncomfortable heartburn. Take your time, eat slowly, and chew your food, no matter how hungry that little baby makes you. Allow some time for digestion, too, before lying down, and that will help. Avoid spicy foods, coffee, and foods with fatty acids. Ginger and chamomile are both good for soothing heartburn.

Constipation

If you are constipated think fiber! Oats, flax seeds, almonds, and fruits and vegetables are all high in fiber. Eating watermelon is a great way to cure constipation because the water in it helps flush food through the bowels. Chamomile tea is another remedy for constipation. It will relax your intestines and make you feel overall relaxed as well.

Swelling

This is quite common during the last few months of pregnancy, especially when the weather is hot and muggy. Swelling can occur around the ankles, calves, hands, feet, wrists, fingers, and face. If swelling occurs, try to avoid eating foods with too much salt, and make sure you drink plenty of water. Foods like celery, apples, watercress and citrus fruits will help you urinate more, which will ultimately help with swelling.

Headaches

Unfortunately, headaches are pretty common during both the first and third trimesters of pregnancy. The easiest way to avoid headaches is to be sure to drink plenty of water (try 8 glasses per day). A cool cloth covering the forehead and eyes will also help. Try to lie in a quiet dark room and get some sleep with the cloth over your eyes. It may be a good idea to ask your doctor about magnesium tablets. Honey and cinnamon have also been known to help with headaches.

Hemorrhoids

Aside from numerous over the counter creams, there are also home remedies that are effective. Apply aloe vera, apple cider vinegar, coconut oil, or witch hazel to the inflamed area with a cotton ball.

Stress Levels

Another way to keep your unborn baby (and yourself) happy is to manage your stress levels. Mindfully managing your stress levels is probably one of the best things you can do. It may not always be easy, but deep breathing during times of extra stress can equalize and give you balance.

Practicing aromatherapy is a great way to destress. These aromatherapy scents can be found as an essential oil or as incense:

- Ylang ylang
- Tea tree
- Sweet orange
- Sandalwood
- Rosewood
- Rose otto
- Petitgrain
- Patchouli
- Neroli
- Mandarin
- Lime
- Lemongrass
- Lemon
- Lavender
- Grapefruit
- Ginger
- Geranium
- Eucalyptus
- Roman Chamomile
- Chamomile
- Bergamot

Prenatal Yoga

Practicing yoga during pregnancy can be beneficial. For instance, it gives you a much-needed energy boost, regulates your nerves, regulates digestion, helps you work through body aches and pains, and prepares your body for labor. Besides, regularly practicing yoga can help to calm a worried mind and help you and baby feel at peace. Obviously, you aren't going to over-do it or over-stretch. Always listen to your body and take it slow.

The Polar Bear

If you're familiar with yoga, this is similar to the Child's Pose. Sit on your knees on a soft, comfortable area of the rug. Spread your knees apart as needed to allow for the baby bump. Bend gently down and place your forearms onto the floor. Your knees should be slightly wider than hip distance apart, but keep your feet as close together as possible. Place your forehead into your arms and relax your body down into the pose. Your baby should be hanging in your belly like a hammock as you stretch. This is a comfortable stretch and can help with opening up the hips during birth. It will take the pressure off your spine and your hips.

Take 5-7 slow, deep breaths and come up out of the pose slowly.

The Wide Squat

Stand with your feet about hip-distance apart. Stand firm and squat down slowly, leaving knees apart to have room for the baby bump. Press your hands together and push out your elbows onto the inner parts of your knees. You should be able to feel the stretching in your inner thighs and up your spine, which will help with relieving tight muscles and back pain.

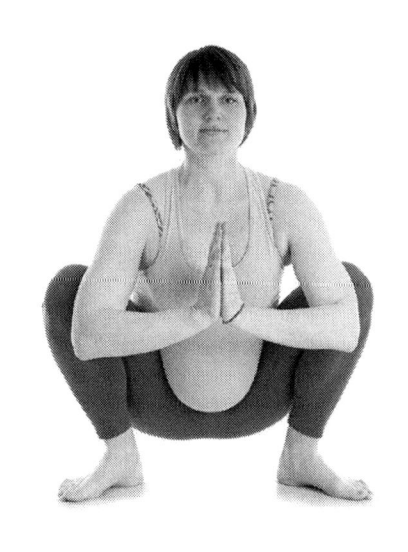

Stretch and breathe steadily for 5-7 breaths and come out of the pose slowly.

Seated Twist

Another way to gently stretch your back is through the seated twist. Sit on the floor with one leg extended and the other leg bent. Obviously, once again, you will need to leave room for the baby. Use the same elbow as the bent knee and gently press against the inside of your knee, keeping your arm bent and your fingertips pointing upward. Place the other arm extended behind you (it should not be too extended, but enough support to comfortably hold you up into the stretch) and gently twist as you turn your head back toward the extended arm.

Do this for 5-7 deep breaths and repeat the same on the other side.

Remember, to enjoy your pregnancy, and embrace of your physical changes. There is another life inside you, so make sure you stay relaxed and keep away from stress. In the next chapter, we shall explore and differentiate the commonly known myths and facts during pregnancy.

Chapter 3
Pregnancy Myths

Chapter 3: Pregnancy Myths

Along with pregnancy comes many myths that have been passed down from generation to generation. Some that have been disproven for many years and some that are simply based on superstition.

Pregnancy can be stressful enough and these myths can cause it to be even more stressful, but that does not have to be. In this chapter, we will go over several common myths that pregnant women have to deal with, and then we will discuss the facts surrounding the myth

Myth 1

Myth- Pregnant women cannot eat sushi.

Fact- Women in Japan have been eating sushi while pregnant for hundreds of years, and there has been no scientific proof that eating raw fish raises the chances of complications in pregnancy. The only thing that you must be aware of is the mercury levels in the fish. It is for this reason that many women avoid eating fish when they are pregnant, but as long as you are eating low mercury level fish, there is no need to avoid your favorite sushi.

Myth 2

Myth- Pregnant women should not exercise.

Fact- For years it was said that pregnant women should avoid exercise as much as possible, but new studies have found that it is not only healthy for the mother to exercise, but it is healthier for the baby as well. It also helps with post-pregnancy weight loss and can make labor easier.

Myth 3

Myth- Pregnant women must gain weight.

Fact- The amount of weight that you need to gain during pregnancy greatly depends on what your pre-pregnancy weight is. For example, a woman who is of normal weight when she becomes pregnant may only need to gain about 20 pounds during her pregnancy. A person who is underweight may need to gain 25 pounds and a person who is overweight may only need to gain 10 pounds.

Myth 4

Myth- Pregnant women should not take baths.

Fact- A pregnant woman can take a bath instead of a shower in order to relax or relieve sore muscles, but the temperature of the water should not be above 98 degrees.

Myth 5

Myth- Pregnancy comes with morning sickness.

Fact- Not all pregnant women will suffer from morning sickness. Each pregnancy is different, and just because you had morning sickness with one, does not mean you will have it with another. It all depends on your hormone levels.

Myth 6

Myth- Pregnant women should not lift anything over their head.

Fact- Pregnant woman are still able to live a normal life, and they can lift objects up to 25 pounds. However a pregnant woman should not be lifting anything over 25 pounds, so make sure you get someone to help you when you want to move the furniture.

Myth 7

Myth- *Walking makes labor go faster.*

Fact- While walking will help to make you feel more comfortable, it has never been proven to make labor move more quickly. There is, in fact, no possible way to make labor go faster than what your body is prepared for. Let the baby come when it is ready, but enjoy those walks to help relieve soreness in the body

There are countless different myths that many people will tell you about pregnancy, from how you are carrying the baby to tell the sex to what you should and should not eat. The truth is, the majority of these are nothing but myths, and if you are unsure, you should talk to your doctor about it.

The most important thing that you can know is that you should continue your life just as you have been living it while you are pregnant. If you were an avid runner before becoming pregnant, by all means continue to run, but it is not advised that you should begin any strenuous workout when you are pregnant.

Many myths about pregnancy are spread around and the problem is that they are just that, myths. We have to educate ourselves about which is fact and which is fiction. In the next chapter, we will explore childbirth options that work for you.

Chapter 4
Childbirth Options That Work for You

Chapter 4: Childbirth Options That Work for You

As a newly pregnant woman, you have a lot to think about and plan for. One of the most important things you will have to explore is which childbirth option is going to best suit your needs and your partner's needs. Here are a few things that might help you take a step in the right direction.

Traditional Hospital Birth

Traditionally, an obstetrician or family practitioner delivers the baby in a hospital. A lot of women who had past complications or medical conditions will most likely take this route, just to be on the safe side.

Midwife

Midwives offer safe delivery and care with more natural approaches and without very much medical intervention. A midwife can deliver in the hospital, birthing centers, or inside the comfort of your own home.

Birthing Centers

Birthing centers offer a more relaxed, less hustle-bustle environment. Some women prefer the freedom of decision making during the labor process, one that is low risk and little intervention.

Home Birth

A midwife is normally present due to the amount of preparation that goes into a home birth. While it can be a comfortable option, unexpected complications can arise. So, it is wise to remain open and plan a hospital visit in case of an emergency.

Cesarean Section

Cesarean Section (also called C-Section) is a routine operation normally used when there are complications with the birth. If the baby is unable to pass through the birth canal properly, this will be the most appropriate option.

Start thinking about what birth plan works best for you. Talk with your doctor or midwife to establish a plan, especially if you are going to choose home birth.

The development of the baby

Ultrasound

Having an ultrasound (also called a sonogram) can be exciting, but it is a necessary step to make sure the baby is growing properly inside you and is moving into position when the time comes closer to the delivery date.

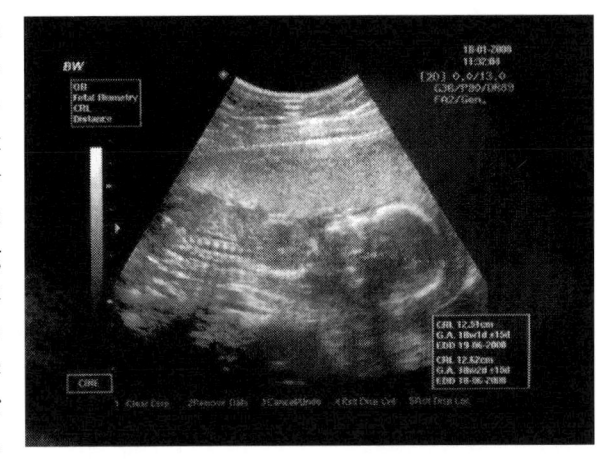

You should also experience a couple of ultrasounds throughout the entire pregnancy to check the health and development of the baby.

There are three different types of ultrasounds. The first, and most commonly known, is the 2D ultrasound. A 2D ultrasound is a white, x-ray-like image, profile of the baby. This 2D imagery shows a flat image of the baby, from all angles, where you can see the baby, the heartbeat, and might be able to tell the gender of the baby.

3D ultrasound is able to produce a 3D image using special software. Instead of a plain white image of your baby, 3D allows you to see more of what the baby will look like. Not only can you tell the gender of the baby, but you are also able to see some facial features.

4D ultrasound improves on 3D ultrasound with a sharper image of the baby and includes a video of the baby's movements and facial expressions. As a matter of fact, this will be the most realistic image of your baby taken before he or she is born. This type of ultrasound requires special equipment and may not be readily available in every office.

First Trimester

The first trimester is week 1 to week 12. The baby appears as an embryo and is only about the size of a kidney bean. The heart will be palpitating quickly and the intestines, eyelids, earlobes, nose, and mouth are all beginning to form. During the first trimester, an ultrasound can confirm the pregnancy, check for the heartbeat, look for abnormalities, make sure the ovaries, cervix, uterus, and placenta are adjusting well, and will determine a due date.

Second Trimester

The second trimester is from week 12 to week 24. The baby is between 3-4 inches long and weighs 1-2 ounces. The fingers and toes are well formed by now and his or her skeleton is forming from cartilage into bone. These are the most exciting weeks because you will feel the baby begin to move around inside you. He or she will also begin to develop the ability to hear. An ultrasound during this time will generally check for appropriate fetus growth, the positioning of the baby, and any abnormalities.

Third Trimester

The third trimester is from week 24 to week 40. During this period, the baby will be able to deposit fat throughout his or her body, weighing at around 3-4 pounds and is probably somewhere near 13 inches. You've gotten used to all the movement, and the baby can now respond to stimulating factors, even inside the womb. The ultrasound during this time period is to check for appropriate positioning of the baby, make sure the baby gets enough oxygen, check for abnormalities, and assure the cervix is at an appropriate length.

Get Ready For Baby!

A great way to ease your mind is to prepare, as much as you can, for the birth of the baby. Just to be sure you don't get overwhelmed, make a preparation checklist, and check things off one at a time. This way, when the baby finally comes, you will be able to relax and rest assured that everything is set in place.

Pelvic exercises

While prenatal yoga exercises will assist with opening up the hips during labor, pelvic exercise can help shorten the first stages of labor as well as pushing time. All you have to do is to squeeze the muscles as if you were trying to stop a flow of urine and hold for ten seconds at a time. Do this about 5 to 8 times once a day.

Set up the baby's room

Sure, you'll get a lot of stuff that the baby isn't going to use right away, so just break it down to the bare essentials: bottles, diapers, burping clothes, newborn clothes that fit, a crib, blankets, and maybe a baby monitor.

Trial run

Another thing that might ease your mind is to pack yours and baby's bag for the hospital visit and make a trial run to the hospital. Make sure to keep the gas tank full during the weeks you are expected to deliver.

Maternity leave

An important part of easing an expecting mother's mind is to get your maternity leave figured out. Talk to your boss about concerns, and finish up any work that might need to be done before you take your leave.

Go shopping

Of course, you will want to spend every last cent on your baby, but don't forget you will need some maternity clothes for the next few months. Consignment shops are great for finding all kinds of styles and sizes.

Schedule doctor appointments

Once you find out you are pregnant, you will need to see the OBGYN. They will most likely schedule you for several check-up appointments throughout your pregnancy.

Going back to work

It's never too early to start planning for childcare for when you go back to work. It's great to have a plan set in place so you're not feeling stressed when it comes closer to time to get back to it.

Baby Shower

You probably won't be the one planning the baby shower now, but you will most likely get the exciting task of choosing items for the registry.

Now, we are all ready to welcome the newborn into this world. In the next chapter, we will highlight what you can expect over the next 30 days after birth.

Chapter 5
What to Expect 30 Days After

Chapter 5: What to Expect 30 Days After

You recognize that your body has gone through dramatic changes during your pregnancy and now it's time to recuperate. The first misconception some may have is that once the baby is gone so will be the baby bump. This is not necessarily true, but don't panic! Your uterus needs time to shrink back down to size. The truth is, most new moms find themselves only about 10-12 pounds lighter after having a 7-8 pound baby. Take the first thirty days to readjust to your new life and heal.

Urinating

If you have trouble urinating after the delivery, a catheter may be put in place to drain your bladder. This is especially true if you have undergone a Cesarean section, as you will most likely have a catheter in place for a few days after delivery. You may not feel the regular urge to urinate right away and find that you can only urinate in small amounts. The good news is that once you are able to urinate with ease over the next few days after having the baby, you will lose another 5 pounds of mostly water weight.

Sweating

Since your body is going to try and get rid of excess water in your system, you will probably find that you break out into sweats often. This only lasts a few days after having the baby.

Skin

Use lotion or cocoa butter on fresh stretch marks to get them to fade. You might want to consider using cocoa butter every day on your baby bump as it grows too, to decrease the number of stretch marks you will have. You may also experience dry skin or dark circles under the eyes. This will fade with time.

Hair Loss

It is common to experience large amounts of hair loss a few weeks after pregnancy. The reason for this is that your average daily hair loss has been interrupted by being pregnant, and now it has to play make catch up. Don't worry, things will return back to normal after a few months.

Back Pain

You will probably have a tight back over the next few weeks while your abdominal muscles are trying to build back up again.

Recognizing Postpartum Depression (PPD)

Experiencing a bout of depression, anxiety, and irritability is sometimes normal for a new mother. It may come on from stress and lack of sleep. If you find that a lot of rest doesn't seem to be helping, you are having severe fits of anger and sadness, or have a drastic change in your appetite PPD is a possible factor.

The best thing you can do is recognize whether or not you have developed these symptoms and talk to someone within your support system. They may have already recognized your strange behavior and expressed concern. It is important to remember that these are normal feelings to experience right after having a baby, and you shouldn't feel ashamed in any way. The important thing is to get help and talk with your loved ones about what is really going on.

How to treat PPD

Symptoms of postpartum depression may come on unexpectedly, but they usually go away with time, especially when you have someone you can trust to talk to. This can be a family member, a partner, your doctor, or a therapist. The next important thing to remember when dealing with PPD is to ask for help with the baby when you are feeling stressed or overwhelmed. Too often, new mothers feel that they have to do everything on their own, but PPD is normal and will subside with time. While you are feeling these symptoms, please ask for help from any support system you might have.

Aside from talking with friends, family, and your OBGYN, take the time to destress yourself. Remember, you just went through 9 months of major changes physically, mentally, and emotionally, and it might take you a few weeks to get back on track. Try some of these natural, safe ways to soothe your mind, body, and spirit.

Eat right

Obviously, when you are eating right, you are getting more vitamins and nutrients than you would if you were eating fatty, processed foods. Try adding these essentials into your daily diet: apples, avocados, beans, blueberries, blackberries, raspberries, strawberries, onions, mushrooms, tomatoes, walnuts, and seeds like sunflower seeds, flax seeds, hemp seeds, and chia seeds.

Exercise

Regular, light exercise increases the levels of serotonin (a natural chemical in the brain that makes you feel good) in your brain. 10 minutes a day can really change your mood and make you feel happy and energized.

Be positive

Mindfully trying to have a positive attitude can alter the way things happen in your life. Do your best to stay positive and find the silver lining in bad situations. Deep, calming breathing during stressful times can often help you see the big picture and let go of more petty things that might upset you. And find some time to laugh and enjoy life! There is a reason they say laughter is the best medicine.

Natural remedies

Aromatherapy is great for treating depression. Using essential oils like bergamot, neroli, eucalyptus, and chamomile will uplift the spirit.

Learn How Babies Communicate

Newborns communicate through cries. This may seem like a foreign language to you at first. But, soon you will discover and learn your baby's language and response to the needs of your little one.

The cries usually indicate something has gone wrong, be it hunger, wet bottom, cold feet, sleepiness, or the need to be held and cuddled. The most common baby's language is:

Short and low-pitched cry– "I am hungry, feed me."

Choppy cry– "I am upset, comfort and cuddle me."

Sometimes the babies can also cry when feeling overwhelmed, be it sights or sounds that are surrounding him or her, for no clear reason.

It is common that newborns cry and show fussiness, especially in the early evening and at midnight. However, it is advisable for you to call your doctor if the cries are prolonged and due to:

The baby is sick. Check the temperature and call the doctor immediately if the temperature hits 100.4°F (38°C) or more.

The baby may be suffering from an eye irritation. This could be due to a scratched cornea or presence of "foreign body" in a baby's eye that is causing irritation.

The baby could be in pain. Check thoroughly if there is an object that could be hurting the baby's skin. For instance, check the diaper pin, any hair tourniquet wrapped around the fingers or toes, etc.

The newborns may develop colic (cry inconsolably) when he or she cries more than 3 hours per day or 3 days per week for 3 weeks. Although this is upsetting, the good news is most newborns outgrow it at around 3 or 4 months of age.

Soothing Newborn Colic

Having a colicky baby can be frustrating when you don't know what to do to help. A lot of times, the baby might just have uncomfortable gas, in which case you can bounce and try to pat the back to help with belching. Another way to help with gas is to lay the baby on its back and gently work the legs in a bicycle motion. This can help airflow and allow gas to release.

Swaddling the baby in a blanket, a walk in the stroller, a ride in the car, and playing slow, soothing music are all things that may pacify a colicky baby. White noise is also a popular way to get baby to calm down because it reminds them of being in the womb. Run the vacuum cleaner, run water from the faucet, or turn on a static station on the radio to emulate this noise (you could also purchase a white noise machine if you find it extremely beneficial). Chamomile, lemon balm, peppermint, and fennel are all safe, calming herbal teas that can be added to the formula to calm the baby.

Hours of sleep for newborn

Newborns do not have a sense of day and night. They sleep round the clock, and because their small stomachs do not hold "food" long enough to satisfy themselves, they wake up often to eat, regardless if it is day or night.

A newborn can sleep up to 18 hours a day in the first months, waking every couple of hours throughout the day to be fed. Breastfed babies need to be fed more often, about every 2 hours or so, as compared to formula fed babies. They tend to feed less often, because it is less digestible, so about every 3 to 4 hours.

It is important that the baby shows good weight gain in the initial first few weeks. Hence, if the baby sleeps for longer stretches, you may need to wake your baby, at least, every 3 hours or so to feed, even at night.

I must say that the first months of a newborn are some of the hardest or most stressful for parents who need to wake up many times to tend to the baby throughout the night. The good news is most babies start to sleep longer through the night (about 4-6 hours

Chapter 6: Breastfeed or Formula Feed

Most of the renowned health organizations—including the American Academy of Pediatrics (AAP), the American Medical Association (AMA), and the World Health Organization (WHO)—recommend breastfeeding as the best choice for babies. The AAP recommends that babies be breastfed exclusively for the first 6 months and encourage longer if both the mother and baby are willing.

Although experts believe breast milk contains the right balance of nutrients for babies, breastfeeding may not be a suitable choice for all mothers due to comfort level, lifestyle, and specific medical conditions. Hence, both mother and baby can have a wonderful experience when you make the right choice between breastfeeding and formula feeding the baby.

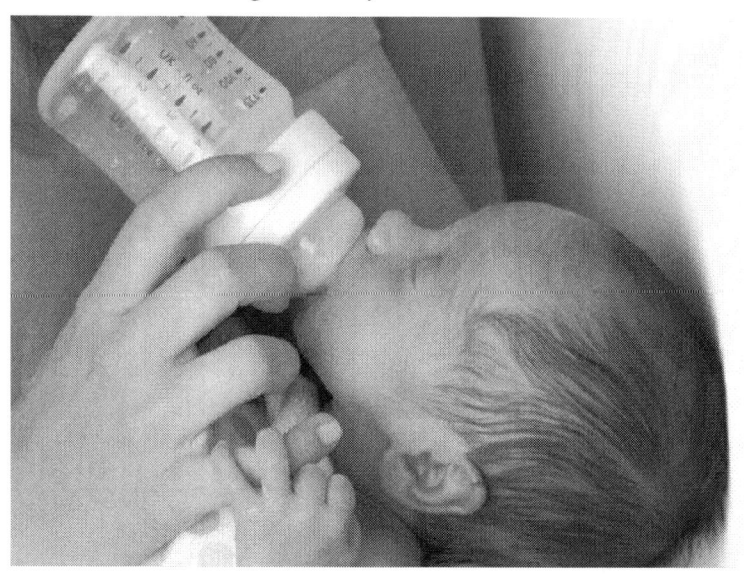

Some mothers fear that breastfeeding is the only way to bond with their baby. The truth is mothers will always create a special bond with their children, regardless if you breastfeed or use formula. Therefore, mothers who give up breastfeeding for whatever reason should not feel guilty, but that they are choosing what is best for them and their child.

All for Breastfeeding

Below there are some highlights of the many benefits of breastfeeding:

Fighting infections and other conditions

Breastfed babies tend to be healthier as compared to the formula-fed babies. This is because breast milk contains antibodies and other germ-fighting factors. These are transferred to a baby to protect and strengthen the immune system, keeping the baby from infections like:

- Cold
- Gastroenteritis
- Ear infections
- Diarrhea
- Respiratory infections
- Meningitis
- Allergies
- Asthma
- Diabetes
- Obesity
- Sudden infant death syndrome (SIDS)

Nutrition and ease of digestion

Breast milk is often named as the "perfect food" for a human baby's digestive system. Its composites include lactose, protein (whey and casein), and fat that are easily digested by a newborn. Hence, breastfed babies have fewer bouts of diarrhea or constipation.

Although, breast milk contains many of the vitamins and minerals that a newborn requires, it does not provide vitamin D—calcium and phosphorus—which is necessary for strong bones. To bridge this shortfall, AAP recommends that all breastfed babies receive vitamin D supplements during the first

2 months, and continue to do so until the baby consumes enough vitamin D

Breast milk is free

Unless you are pumping breast milk where you need to pay for bottles, nipples, and other supplies, breast milk itself does not cost you a cent. However, most will need to pay for formula (unless you work in companies that manufacture formula and they give it away as part of the employee benefits). Because of the fact that breastfed babies are stronger in their immune system, this also means you will need fewer trips to the doctor and less money will be spent on prescriptions and over-the-counter medicines.

Cultivate different tastes

A nursing mother would need extra calories together with a wide variety of foods and well-balanced diet. Therefore, babies are being introduced to different flavors via their mothers' breast milk. This will cultivate the babies to be more acceptable to "familiar tasting" solid foods thereafter.

Convenience

The availability of breast milk has no restriction on the venue, is always fresh, and comes with the right temperature and composition. There is no concern of sterilizing bottles and nipples, checking the temperature and composition of milk, and making milk mixtures in the middle of the night.

Smarter babies

Many researchers have also suggested that exclusively breastfed children tend to have higher IQs than those who were formula-fed.

"Skin-to-skin" contact

Many mothers enjoy the unique bonding experience with their babies while nursing. The close encounter of skin-to-skin contact enhances the physical and emotional connection between the mother and the baby. Hormones, such as prolactin, are released and create a peaceful, nurturing sensation that allows both mother and baby to relax, and oxytocin, which promotes a strong sense of love and bonding between the two. Besides, the baby will feel more secure, which is important for the wellbeing and development, when he or she hears the mother's heartbeat, breathing, and familiar, soothing voice during breastfeeding.

Beneficial for the mother

To produce enough healthy milk, nursing mothers are advised to eat a healthy and well-balanced diet, drink lots of fluids and have plenty of rest. Since breastfeeding burns calories and shrinks the uterus, it helps the mother to slim down to her pre-pregnancy shape and weight faster. Studies also show that breastfeeding helps to reduce the risk of breast and ovarian cancer, high blood pressure, diabetes, cardiovascular disease, and uterine and rheumatoid arthritis.

Breastfeeding Challenges

Breastfeeding can be easy for some mothers, but it will take some time for others to master the technique and routine of breastfeeding.

Some of the concerns of new mothers, especially during the first few weeks, may include:

Personal comfort

Initially, some mothers may feel uncomfortable with breastfeeding. But with proper education, support, and practice, most mothers overcome this.

Latch-on pain

This is normal initially (up to first 10 days) and lasts for a minute or two during each feeding. It is recommended that the nursing mothers seek help from a lactation consultant or doctor if the breastfeeding hurts throughout the nursing, or the nipples and/or breast are sore, in case of infection. But more often, it's got to do with proper technique.

Time and frequency of feedings

Breastfeeding demands substantial time commitment from a mother, particularly in the initial period when babies need to be fed often. Breast milk is digested faster than formula, leading to a demand from the newborn every 2 or 3 hours in the first few weeks. This may pose a challenge for a working mother, or when she is running errands or traveling.

Diet

Mothers who are breastfeeding their babies need to be extra conscious of their diet since the food can be passed to the baby through the breast milk. For instance, if the nursing mother drinks alcohol or consumes caffeine drink, a small amount can pass to the baby through breast milk. To eliminate this transfer, breastfeeding should take place at least 2 hours after each single alcoholic drink; and caffeine intake should be limited to a maximum of 300 milligrams (about one to three cups of regular coffee) per day. These will aid to prevent potential issues like restlessness and irritability in some babies. Similar to the diet during pregnancy, a nursing mother should not eat fish that are high in mercury.

Maternal medical conditions and medicines

Mothers with medical conditions such as HIV or AIDS or those involved in chemotherapy or with certain medicines and breast surgery should check with the doctor or a lactation consultant to make sure breastfeeding is safe before proceeding to nurse your baby. It is also advisable to check with the doctor about the safety of taking existing or potential medicines while breastfeeding.

All for Formula Feeding

Infant formula is a healthy alternative for mothers who are unable to breastfeed due to medical reasons, or who decide not to due to lifestyle or other reasons.

The U.S. Food and Drug Administration (FDA) regulates formula companies to ensure they provide all the necessary nutrients for babies to grow and thrive. Most of them even contain vitamins (vitamin D) that are lacking in breast milk.

The formula also supports babies who have typical dietary requirements. For an instant, a special formula will be needed for the baby who has special nutritional needs.

Below is a list of other reasons mothers choose to formula feed:

Convenience and flexibility

Mothers can offload some of the feeding duties to her partner or caregiver with a bottle (this is also true for nursing mothers who pump their breast milk). Moms can be far less stressed and dad can get more engaged in the feeding process and create a bond with the baby too. There is no need to look for a private place to nurse in public for formula-feeding mothers. Also, the mother would not be required to reschedule work or other obligations and activities during feeding time.

Time and frequency of feedings

Since breast milk is more easily digestible than formula, there will be less feeding required for formula-fed babies as compared to breastfeeding babies.

Diet

Mothers that choose to formula feed have much less concern on their diet. What they consumed will not be passed to their babies through breast milk.

Formula Feeding Challenges

Mothers should take the following into consideration when opting to formula feed their babies.

Lack of antibodies

Breast milk contains antibodies and immunity-boosting properties and is uniquely produced by the mother for her baby. The commercial formulas are yet to duplicate the complexity of breast milk, lacking the added protection against infections and illness for a baby as compared to breast milk.

Planning and organization

Unlike breast milk, which is available 24/7 and served at the right temperature, mothers who opt for formula need to do some planning and organizing to make sure that the formula does not run out of stock. They also have to make sure they have the necessary supplies to clean and sterilize bottles and nipples, and all of this needs to be easily accessible and ready to go when making each bottle. Poor hygiene often leads to nasty infections. Parents also can be overwhelmed and stressed if they have a very hungry and fussy baby to attend to especially in the middle of the night.

Expense

The formula can be costly, and it may cost as much as $1,500 during the first year. Unlike breast milk, which is freely produced by the mother, the formula needs to be purchased. Among them, special formulas (such as soy) cost much more than basic powdered formula.

The possibility of producing gas and constipation

Because the formula is less digestible as compared to breast milk, formula-fed babies tend to produce more gas and suffer from more constipation than breastfed babies.

How you are going to feed your newborn can be quite a challenging decision to make. Regardless, mothers should not be judged about their feeding decision, as they do have the right to choose what they think is best for them and their baby. However, I would strongly encourage them to seek as much information as possible from their health care providers, so they will come to a decision based on the facts and what is best for their family.

Bonus Material

Bonus Material: Step-By-Step Guide to Successful Breastfeeding

The most important thing that will make your breastfeeding sessions successful is to find the right position for both you and baby. In order for a baby to latch on, you should both be relaxed and comfortable. Comfort means putting your feet up, propping up your arms with pillows, and propping baby with pillows.

When your baby is hungry, he or she will instinctively turn its head toward your breast. Once it is time to eat, try one of the positions listed below to see which works best.

The Cradle

In the cradle hold, rest the baby's head in the crook of your elbow and pull in close so your bellies are facing, even touching, one another. Raise the baby up with your arm until it latches on. Place a pillow under your arm and baby for comfortable propping purposes.

The Cross Cradle

Hold the baby's body in the crook of your other arm while supporting the head with your hand and guiding it into latching on. Again, use supporting pillows for the best comfort.

The Football

Using the same side for both the arm and breast, cradle the baby's body in your arm and support its head with your hand. This is a popular position with women who have had a C-section because the baby doesn't have to lie across the abdomen.

Sideways

Lying down on your side, get baby propped up with a pillow or prop him or her up with your arm. Baby can lie on its side, too, while it eats.

So, how do you get a baby to latch on properly? First, encourage your baby to open wide by placing your nipple on the mouth. Then, roll the under part of your breast down into the baby's mouth, causing it to open wider. Once your nipple reaches into the baby's mouth, it will be able to latch on and will begin to instinctively suckle. When the baby is feeding properly, you will feel a tingling sensation and you should hear the baby gulping. If the baby seems unsettled and its suckling is causing you pain, you may want to try to re-latch because it may not be getting any milk. Hearing a clicking sound while feeding could indicate that only air is getting through. Also, baby's cheeks should be nice and full and not sunken in.

Drink lots of water when nursing to help produce more milk, and avoid caffeine as much as possible, as this will make your baby restless. The first couple of days after delivery you might experience engorgement, which means your breasts can become sore, hard, and tender. The best way to avoid engorgement is to start breastfeeding as soon as possible and as often as possible to relieve the pressure.

Engorgement

Engorgement can be extremely uncomfortable and at times it can be difficult, or even painful, to breastfeed. To ease the pressure and pain, place a warm compress on your breasts a couple of minutes before you begin feeding. This will help get the milk flowing. Do not apply the compress for more than 3 minutes, as it could have an adverse effect.

Once feeding begins, you can massage the breast the baby is feeding on to relieve some pressure and tightness. Cold packs can help with swelling and the uncomfortable feeling, but only use them for about ten minutes at a time. You can also use a breast pump to relieve some of the pressure, but too much pumping can lead to producing more milk, which will encourage engorgement for a longer period of time. A lot of times, wearing a supportive nursing bra can help, especially during the night. Make sure it doesn't have the underwire in it, as that can be too restricting. Aspirin and Ibuprofen can help with the discomfort and both are safe to use when you are nursing.

Common Fears

A lot of women fear that they will not be able to produce enough milk for the baby. This fear may come from not physically being able to control the amount of milk actually produced. The fact of the matter is just be sure to drink lots of water, and even if your milk production slows down after a while, you will always be able to catch up.

Other times, there is a concern that the baby should spend a certain amount of time on each breast. Just do what the baby wants here and allow him or her to feed where most comfortable. Your body produces on a supply and demand, as needed basis.

Another common fear is of feeding the baby when you are sick. You won't have to worry about passing over an illness through your milk. Your milk has strong antibodies in it that will actually help ward off any illnesses for the baby. If you stop feeding during a period of time when you are ill, it is a possibility that your milk supply will slightly decrease if the baby isn't feeding. The same can be said if you are on medication. Due to the antibodies in the milk, you being on medication will not affect the baby through feeding.

Premature babies may take a little longer to latch onto the breast, but they are the ones who can most definitely benefit from the mother's natural milk. The main reason for this is because it contains essential nutrients necessary for the baby to grow at a healthy rate.

Breast pump

When it may be time for you to go out for a night or get back to work, or just to give yourself a break, breast pumps not only allow you to continue producing enough milk but also to store some for later. You will need to massage the breast and try to remain relaxed to make pumping a lot easier. It may seem strange to you at first, but using a pump can give you a real break and will get more comfortable the more you use it.

It's true that most women produce more milk first thing in the morning, so keep that in mind if you are pumping to store any. Also, you can use a pump anywhere from 30-60 minutes after actually feeding. You may be reluctant to feed right after using the pump, but you can do this as well. If you are planning on feeding your baby breast milk but use only the bottle, be prepared to pump 8-10 times per day.

Once you and baby are able to connect during these feeding sessions, there will truly be no other comparison. Even when the baby is having a tough time latching on, keep at it and keep trying.

Conclusion

The fact is you will probably get plenty of advice from relatives, strangers, and friends on pregnancy and new motherhood, but all the choices you make are ultimately up to you. Get as much advice as you can and talk to the support system around you and people you trust.

You will need to find a balanced diet for yourself and your unborn child. Do your best to take advantage of organic foods rather than processed foods, and ask your doctor about holistic approaches rather than pharmaceutical approaches. Research natural remedies as well as medicinal remedies that work, and be sure to do daily light exercises, especially yoga practices, in order to enhance a smooth delivery.

When you begin to feel overwhelmed, make your list of things to do. Get the baby's room ready, decide where and how you would like to give birth and secure emergency plans with your spouse and family. Take your daily tasks one day at a time and watch it all come together. Once the baby is born, everything will be set into place and you can be ready for as much bonding time as you need.

Whenever someone tells you that you should not eat something, should not do something, or that you should do something that you are not doing, make sure that you take the time to research it or ask your doctor. So many myths about pregnancy are spread around and the problem is that they are just that, myths.

Now that you have a list of appropriate foods and a list of remedies for common ailments, you should be well on your way to a healthy and enjoyable pregnancy. You should also have the tools you need to help with a colicky baby and successful breastfeeding techniques. Not everything can be predictable when expecting a baby, but knowing the basics definitely helps.

After reading this book, you should also be equipped to handle the first thirty days as a new mother. Allow your body to recuperate, but keep in mind that you may continue to experience mood swings, over-sensitivity, or moments of stress or anger. Be aware of the symptoms of PPD and talk to a professional if you think you are experiencing it. Be sure to surround yourself with supportive people and stay as far away from stress as you can. On the flip side, make sure you get the rest you deserve, during both pregnancy and the first thirty days after delivery.

I hope you enjoyed this eBook and have benefited from it. If you did, please leave a review on Amazon.

-- Christie Knight

Printed in Great Britain
by Amazon